MW01490666

# The Daniel Sugar Diet Cookbook

# Get Rid of Sugar Fat & Reduce Blood Pressure in 21 Days!!!

Diabetes Edition

Disclaimer

Table of Contents

Table of Contents

What is the Daniel Sugar Diet?.................6
Why is the Daniel Fast so effective?.........8
Benefits of the Daniel Sugar Diet ...........9
The Daniel Sugar Diet Food List............11
Daily Devotions ...................................13
  Day 1: Sanctification.........................13
  Day 2: Finding Wisdom and Knowledge........15
  Day 3: The Value of Privacy................17
  Day 4: Matthew 6:5-8.......................19
  Day 5: Dealing With Temptation............21
  Day 6: Fueling With The Word Of God.......23
  Day 7: Strength in Weakness...............25
  Day 8: Climbing Mountains.................27
  Day 9: Spiritual Nourishment..............29
  Day 10: A New Comfort Food................31
  Day 11: Self-Control......................33
  Day 12: Self-Control, Part 2.............35
  Day 13: Think About These Things.........37
  Day 14: Being Still Before The Lord......39
  Day 15: Being God's Captive..............41
  Day 16: Cravings.........................43
  Day 17: Worship..........................45
  Day 18: The Big Box......................47
  Day 19: Serving The Boss.................49
  Day 20: Crossing The Finish Line.........51
  Day 21: Mind Renewal.....................53
Breakfast ........................................55

Currant and Almond Toasted Muesli..............55
Stuffed Breakfast Squash............................56
Baked Quinoa.........................................58
Peanut Butter Cakes.................................59
Breakfast Burritos...................................60

Lunch Recipes ........................................61
Veggie Delight........................................61
Sunflower Strawberry Salad.........................62
Garlic and Tomato Soup.............................63
Roasted Broccoli and Asparagus..................64
Marinated Vegetable Salad.........................65
Asian Spinach Salad.................................66
Spicy Black Bean Burgers...........................67
Italian-style Rice and Beans.......................69
Squash and Fennel Soup.............................70
Spring Salad..........................................71
Shining Carrot Soup.................................72
Moo Shu Vegetables.................................73

Dinner................................................74
Grilled Farmer's Market Veggies..................74
Iowa Corn Soup.......................................76
7-Veggie Stew........................................77
Baked Beans..........................................78
Mexican Casserole...................................79
Stuffed Cabbage.....................................81
White Bean Chili.....................................83
"Carmelized" Lentils.................................84
Standard Stir-Fry....................................85
Butternut Squash and Greens.......................86
Roasted Brussels Sprouts and Pomegranate
Dressing...............................................87
Fake-Out Minestrone................................88
Baked Spaghetti Squash.............................89

Indian Chickpeas.......................................91
Conclusion.................................................93

What is the Daniel Sugar Diet?

The Daniel Sugar Diet was developed from the very successful and effective, the **Daniel Fast**. The word *fast* indicates a period of abstinence, usually involving food or drink, for religious and spiritual purposes.

The Daniel fast is a specific type of fast based on scriptures from the book of Daniel, an Old Testament prophet. This particular fast is a *partial fast*, where participants consume a restricted diet.

We use the power and successful techniques of the Daniel Fast and combine it with recipes that specifically cater to individuals with diabetes, high blood pressure, and high cholesterol. This combination releases the effective power of both techniques which provides each individual with amazing life changing results.

This book is FULL OF RECIPES that covers breakfast, lunch, and dinner as you complete your 21 DAY journey to health and feeling better than you ever have. There are 31 unique recipes in total to provide variety so that you can stay motivated through your diet.

Also in this book, we have provided our Christian readers with 21 days of daily devotions to follow as a bonus to further help you on your journey to health. These devotions can be used by everyone in their own individual way.

Why is the Daniel Fast so effective?

It's important to keep in mind that the Daniel Fast is a fast, not just a diet plan. Fasting has been around since ancient times, as evidenced throughout the entirety of the Bible.
Additionally, there are certain health benefits to fasting:

- You rid your body of toxins
- You develop healthier eating habits
- You can lower high blood pressure
- You eventually curb your cravings towards healthier food items

The Daniel Fast is particularly effective because it is, in fact, a partial fast. You select from a host of fruits, vegetables, whole grains, legumes, and seasoning with to build you new diet. By eliminating added sweeteners, you can not only modify your sweet tooth, but also control your blood sugar better. Ridding your plate of solid fats and other animal products will reduce your cholesterol and help your cardiovascular system.

Please consult your doctor before undertaking any radical changes to your diet, such as the Daniel Fast / The Daniel Sugar Diet. Every individual is different and your doctor would be your source for the most accurate information.

Benefits of the Daniel Sugar Diet

The benefits of the Daniel Sugar Diet are endless. The effectiveness of this 21 day diet does surpass a lot of diets as far as health benefits.

Benefits reported from the Daniel Sugar Diet includes (but not limited to):

- Increased energy
- Decreased blood pressure
- Diabetes improving (insulin levels dropping by as much as 23%)
- Improvement in Hypoglycemia
- Weight loss
- Skin improved
- No more bloating
- Improved digestion
- And the list goes on...

Whether we are always aware or not, toxins are always around us and it is virtually impossible not to come in contact with toxins while you go about your daily routine. The air is polluted, the food is not 100% natural or has been enhanced in some way, and water isn't always as innocent as it appears either.

Whether you are completing this 21 day diet to lose weight, to improve and potentially get rid of your diabetes or just to live a more fulfilling and healthy life, the Daniel Sugar Diet will get you to where you want and need to be.

The Daniel Sugar Diet Food List

While being on a diet itself isn't an easy task, knowing what to avoid on the Daniel Sugar Diet is—keep the following guidelines in mind.

**Don't** eat it if it contains:

- Any kind of animal products
- Any kind of dairy whatsoever
- Added sweeteners of any kind (including stevia and honey)
- Leavened bread (Ezekiel bread is even out—it contains sweeteners)
- Food additives, including but not limited to artificial colors, flavorings, and preservatives
- White rice and white flour
- Deep-fried foods of any kind
- Solid fats like margarine, shortening, any kind of Crisco or lard

Here's what you **can** have on the Daniel Fast:

- Water (this is the only beverage you are allowed)
- All fruits and vegetables, be them fresh, frozen, dried/dehydrated, canned, or jarred
- Any and all peas, beans, and nuts, be them fresh, canned, or dried

- Whole grains like whole wheat, brown rice, quinoa, oats, etc.
- Good-quality oils
- Tofu
- Rice cakes
- Unbuttered popcorn
- Natural nut butters
- Vinegar
- Herbs
- Spices
- Salt
- Pepper
- Tofu

Daily Devotions

Day 1: Sanctification

**1 Thessalonians 5:23-24**
*May God himself, the God of peace, sanctify*
*you through and through. May your whole spirit,*
*soul and body be kept blameless at the coming*
*of our Lord Jesus Christ.* The one who calls you is
faithful, and he will do it.

What is sanctification? Many consider it the
process of being made holy. While we may not
be fully sanctified until we are one with Christ, we
take small steps towards becoming more Christ-
like while here on earth.

The discipline of fasting is one of spiritual
disciplines believers practice in order to grow
closer to God; in the process, we become more
like Christ—at least this is our hope, since we are
not completely free from sin. Fasting is one of the
ways to keep your "body...blameless" as stated
in 1 Thessalonians.

Church activities like singing in the choir,
volunteering with the youth group, planning and
participating in Bible studies—these are all have
their place as things we do to help grow and
encourage the fellowship of believers.
Sometimes, however, the social nature of these

activities can distract us from the reason the activity exists in the first place. The difference between fasting and these is that fasting takes place solo. It's just you, one-on-one with God, committing to making small sacrifices in order to grow spiritually in Him.

Though it may seem like a painstaking process, initially, remember that "the one who calls you is faithful." God will be by your side this entire duration of fasting, at the ready whenever you need Him, and He's looking forward to spending more time with you.

*Dear Lord, thank You for being there for me always. Show me ways that I can use this period of fasting to be more like Christ, and help me to stay faithful to this commitment.*

## Day 2: Finding Wisdom and Knowledge

Colossians 2:2-3 (NIV)

*I want them to be encouraged and knit together by strong ties of love. I want them to have complete confidence that they understand God's mysterious plan, which is Christ himself. In him lie hidden all the treasures of wisdom and knowledge.*

In this digital age, it's easy to just flip open your phone or get on the laptop and look up the answers to any question that pops into your mind:

"What time is the movie playing?"
"Is the salon open on Mondays?"
"What is it that makes a diet vegan?"
"Why did the government pass that bill?"

Surely, modern conveniences provide us with information to address both the mundane and the complex aspects of life alike, but the Internet doesn't address the deepest questions of our lives—and it doesn't have to.

Paul writes to the church in Colossus to encourage believers that not only does God have a plan, but also He has revealed that plan to us through Jesus Christ, in who lies "all the treasures of wisdom and knowledge." We don't need the Internet to give us the answers to our biggest questions of our lives because the truth is found in Christ.

Even though it isn't easy in the beginning, fasting is one of the most wonderful ways to allow God to enter your life and speak in notable way. When we make room for Him, He moves in, speaking to us in ways that only He can.

*Dear Lord, help me to use this time of fasting to fully hear your truth, wisdom, and knowledge. Amen.*

Day 3: The Value of Privacy

Matthew 6: 16-18 (NLT)

*"And when you fast, don't make it obvious, as the hypocrites do, for they try to look miserable and disheveled so people will admire them for their fasting. I tell you the truth, that is the only reward they will ever get. But when you fast, comb your hair and wash your face. Then no one will notice that you are fasting, except your Father, who knows what you do in private. And your Father, who sees everything, will reward you.*

If you Google your name, there's a strong chance that you'll find your name, address, LinkedIn page, pictures of your family vacation, and a host of other bits of personal information floating around out there in cyberspace—unless you don't participate in social media or you have set very strict privacy filters. Usually, that's not the case: we live in a world that is more connected now then ever, and even the word "connected" has become its own buzzword of sorts.

The church is not immune to promoting a lack of privacy. While there is something to be said for building connections, there is also great value in privacy, namely the privacy of our spiritual selves before the Lord. There are many churches who participate in a Daniel Fast together as a way to encourage members, spur on spiritual growth, and prepare themselves for worship or a time of great change within the church—all tremendous benefits. However, it benefits us most to keep in mind the rules and regulations regarding fasting that came from the God's Own Son Himself.

Jesus teaches that when we're fasting, we should continue to take care of ourselves and not let the effects of hunger and exhaustion come over us. More importantly, he stresses that nobody should really know that we are fasting "except your Father, who knows what you do in private." A quick peek through the New Testament reveals that Jesus was a big fan of keeping the details of your personal relationship with God personal, and it's no surprise that His view on fasting is no different.

When you find yourself challenged by your fast, don't rush to blog, tweet, or tell a friend about it. Bring your struggles right into the lap of the Lord of comfort and healing.

*Dear Lord, as I fast, help me to turn to You and You alone in times of discouragement and struggles so that I may receive the many blessings You have in store for me.*

Day 4: Matthew 6:5-8

*And when you pray, you must not be like the hypocrites. For they love to stand and pray in the synagogues and at the street corners, that they may be seen by others. Truly, I say to you, they have received their reward. But when you pray, go into your room and shut the door and pray to your Father who is in secret. And your Father who sees in secret will reward you. "And when you pray, do not heap up empty phrases as the Gentiles do, for they think that they will be heard for their many words. Do not be like them, for your Father knows what you need before you ask him.*

We hear many sermons on the importance of fellowship and the communion of the saints. These lessons teach worthy aspects of the Christian life, and they should not be dismissed. After all, we are instructed to help each other, to lean on one another, and to lift each other up in encouragement and prayer. It can be tempting to want to share the joys and struggles of your Daniel Fast with other believers, especially those who are also embarking on this journey of fasting.

However, at this point, you are still in the trenches of your fast, with only a few days remaining. Any struggles or challenges presented to you today and in the days to come should be brought before the Lord and in private, as He commands in this passage from the Sermon on the Mount. Also bear in mind that not only does He request that we come to him one-on-one, but that we refrain from wordiness or "empty phrases." Remember, God knows what is on your heart. All He asks is that we come to Him for guidance, support, and help.

*Dear Lord, help me to stay focused on You and You alone during the remainder of my fasting journey. You know my heart and its desires and struggles. Grant me your peace, patience, guidance, and support as I continue to seek You during this time.*

Day 5: Dealing With Temptation

Luke 4:1-2

*Then Jesus, full of the Holy Spirit, returned from the Jordan River. He was led by the Spirit in the wilderness, where he was tempted by the devil for forty days. Jesus ate nothing all that time and became very hungry.*

As you enter the third day of your Daniel fast, you're probably becoming uncomfortable and irritable—this is to be expected, as you are getting rid of the toxins in your body. Because of this, you might be tempted to "cheat" on your fast, or give the whole thing entirely—and end up feeling even worse in the end for not fulfilling the goal you set out for yourself.

Bring your troubles to Jesus. After all, He knows hunger, and He understands more than anyone, since He Himself was tempted for forty days straight by none other than Satan. He was stranded in the wilderness and ate nothing. The Bible even says that He was "very hungry."

Now, we're not sitting in the middle of the desert wilderness, and we're not fasting for forty days— and we're definitely not Jesus. A partial fast is hard, for sure, but keep in mind that you're still allowed to consume a wide variety of nutritious and tasty fruits and vegetables—more than our Savior was permitted during His fast.

*Dear Lord, humble me during my moments of weakness. Remind me of the temptation that You faced and bless me with the courage to persevere during this tempting time. Let me hold onto Your strength.*

Day 6: Fueling With The Word Of God

Matthew 4: 4 (ESV)

*But he answered, "It is written, "'Man shall not live by bread alone, but by every word that comes from the mouth of God.*

Working hard throughout the day can take a physical and mental toll on a person. This is probably why somebody invented the coffee break: some of us start losing energy right before lunch time, while others find their mid-day slump hitting right around three or four in the afternoon.

We tend to rely on that coffee break, that caffeine, that snack, or even the just that time away from our desks to refresh ourselves before heading back to the grind.

While you are most certainly allowed to have a healthy snack (within the guidelines) throughout this fast, imagine how much more of an impact God could make during this time if you feast on His word prior to each meal? After all, Jesus tells us it is more than food that will sustain us—it is the truth and wisdom contained in scripture and in our communion with the Lord. This is what will get us to the good spots and through the hard spots of life; this is what Jesus sees as equally essential as food.

Consider filling that coffee break with a short Bible study, a time of prayer and meditation, or verse memorization while you are fasting.

*Dear Lord, I know that Your word is just as essential to my life as food. Fill me up with Your truth, Your presence, and Your Holy Spirit.*

Day 7:  Strength in Weakness

2 Corinthians 12: 10 (NLT)

*That's why I take pleasure in my weaknesses, and in the insults, hardships, persecutions, and troubles that I suffer for Christ. For when I am weak, then I am strong.*

Imagine that you haven't set foot in a gym in quite some time—or ever.  You hit the treadmill, the elliptical, and the bike, then you head into the weight room for a little strength training. Your muscles ache and you feel a bit burned out, but you're sure a hot shower, some water, and a good night's sleep will fix that. After all, it's been a while, right?

You plan to take off the next day, following the advice of fitness gurus, but when you're scheduled to hit the gym again, your body just can't bear the thought of it—lifting your arm to brush your teeth was enough for your poor biceps this morning.  However, the experts are right, and you plunge forward into swimming laps in the pool, running a mile, and doing some sit-ups.

What happens to our bodies after some time away from a workout routine isn't so different than what happens after a slew of hard days at the office, drama with family or friends, or any other kind of mental or emotional exhaustion. Nobody enjoys feeling like the world is on their shoulders and they're about to collapse from the immensity of it all.

When times like these arise, even simple habits, tasks, and chores seem to bear more weight. Cracking open your Bible or kneeling in prayer before the Lord—*yeah, right,* you might say. *Not today.* It just feels like one more thing to do that requires so much—and you feel like you've got nothing left.

It is during these times that the apostle Paul writes of his greatest strengths. He's not bragging here, but he's trying to encourage other followers of Jesus: when you're at your weakest and you put out an act of faith where you're still seeking God, you become strong. Seek Him each time you feel weak and you exercise, tone, and build that faith muscle.

*Dear Lord, I want to have a strong faith in You. Please bless my willing spirit and give me the energy I need to spend more time seeking You and knowing You.*

Day 8: Climbing Mountains

Hebrews 12: 28-29 (NIV)

Therefore, since we are receiving a kingdom that cannot be shaken, let us be thankful, and so worship God acceptably with reverence and awe, *for our "God is a consuming fire."*

If you've ever hiked up a mountain, you understand both the joy and the physical anguish that accompany the hike: you know that the trek can be arduous but beautiful, and that views from the summit will be worth the sweat, the pain, and the muscle strain.

Perhaps you have felt like you were climbing two different mountains this week: the mountain of joy—knowing that you would be building your relationship with God during this fast—and the mountain of uncertainty—wondering if you could really do it, if you were cut out for this fasting stuff.

Hebrews 12 talks about the mountain of fear and the mountain of joy. As believers, we have come to the mountain of joy and are not "trembling with fear" (v. 21). We serve a God who presides over a "kingdom that cannot be shaken."

Fasting provides us with ample opportunities for prayer, meditation, reflection, and worship. As we are climbing this mountain of joy, we certainly don't consume as much or as varied foodstuffs, but we can be consumed with fervor and love for God instead.

*Dear Lord, I know that you are a consuming fire. Fill me with your Holy Spirit and your love so that I can climb the mountain of joy and be a light to others.*

Day 9: Spiritual Nourishment

James 1: 19-21 (ESV)

*Know this, my beloved brothers: let every person be quick to hear, slow to speak, slow to anger; for the anger of man does not produce the righteousness of God. Therefore put away all filthiness and rampant wickedness and receive with meekness the implanted word, which is able to save your souls.*

As you enter the seventh day of the fast, you are in the throes of depleting your body of toxins and re-introducing yourself to life-giving food that nourishes your entire system. You might start feeling more energetic and have a greater sense of concentration and alertness.

Just the same way that you are feeding your body a feast of nutritious foods, we can nourish ourselves spiritually by spending time with the Lord and studying scripture.
Doing so will help those scriptures take root in your heart; James refers to it as, "the implanted word."

As you get rid of all the "bad" stuff, food-wise, you can begin to put away the other "bad stuff," like instant reactions, thoughtless speech, taking things personally, and anger-related issues. Over time, you will find those behaviors being replaced with godly behaviors. It is completely possible to do this through God's help and guidance, which is "able to save" our souls! Surely, if God is capable of saving our souls, He can bring us to a place of peace, patience, and calmness in our lives by showing us what changes we need to make.

*Dear Lord, I trust You. I believe that You can replace the negative with the positive, and that Your Word can take root in my heart. Show me what changes I can make in my life to please You.*

Day 10: A New Comfort Food

1 Timothy 6: 6-8 (NIV)

*But godliness with contentment is great gain. For we brought nothing into the world, and we can take nothing out of it. But if we have food and clothing, we will be content with that.*

At the end of a long day, there can sometimes be nothing better than sitting down to a warm meal comprised of your favorite comfort foods. You will find those long days still take place during your Daniel Fast, and it can be challenging to not give into the temptation to make a meal of your non-Daniel-Fast favorites.

However, the Bible helps us to put things in perspective. While the above scripture reference goes on to warn against the love of money, monetary wealth, and material things, it begins by talking about godliness and contentment in the most basic of things. Truly, the foods permitted during this fast are among the most basic, and many do not qualify towards the common idea of "comfort foods."

Still, we are called to be thankful and content, even blessed, because our basic needs are met. Did you wake this morning with a roof over your head, in a comfortable bed? Were you able to put together a morning meal to satisfy the hunger pangs of going without food throughout the night? Do you have clothes to wear to cover you and keep you warm? You are already a step ahead of the game compared to many.

As you go forward into your day, remember to be thankful for what you *do* have and what you *can* eat. This leads you one step closer to godliness.

*Dear Lord, thank You for all that You have given me. Forgive me for any lack of gratitude within my heart. Help me to find contentment in what You have given me so that I may grow closer to you.*

Day 11: Self-Control

Galatians 5:22-23 (NIV)

*But the fruit of the Spirit is love, joy, peace, forbearance, kindness, goodness, faithfulness, gentleness and self-control. Against such things there is no law.*

When you visit an orchard, you can see that the apple trees are well taken care of. Someone has planted those seeds, watered the plant, fed it the proper nutrients, pruned the branches, and watched it blossom. All of this nurturing leads to a healthy plant, one that produces the sweet, juicy, and crispy, crunchy apples that we all enjoy.

Like the farmer tending his orchard, so it is when we allow God to tend our hearts.

When we make room for God in our hearts, and when we dedicate time to getting to know Him, changes start happening within our lives. We find ourselves calmer, happier; we treat others better. We turn to Him in times of trouble, and hold on to the belief that He will bring us through it if He brought us to it. We also experience a greater sense of self-control over our actions and reactions.

It takes strength, dedication, faith, and self-control to live well, and these attributes are especially necessary during a time of fasting. If you want to see the fruit of the Spirit abundant in your life, you need to allow the Holy Spirit to dwell in you, speak to you, and listen in return.

*Dear Lord, I want to bear the fruits of Your Holy Spirit. Dwell in me so that I may be aware of Your voice and leadings, and help me to hear You and be obedient to Your will.*

## Day 12: Self-Control, Part 2

Proverbs 25: 27-28 (NIV)

*It is not good to eat too much honey,*
*nor is it honorable to search out matters that are*
*too deep.*
*Like a city whose walls are broken through*
*is a person who lacks self-control.*

Sometimes we just can't stop ourselves: we decided it's perfectly all right to watch a few more hours of television, play around online for the rest of the night, eat an entire package of Oreos, or spend more money than we planned on a shopping trip. We oftentimes become adept at rationalizing, and can excuse away anything that we may have done in excess:

"It's my birthday, so I can do whatever I want!"
"I had a really long day at work, so I'm entitled to (fill in the blank)."
"I haven't (fill in the blank) in a really long time, so it's ok."

We wind up defending our choices not just to others, but also to ourselves. The problem here isn't the *what*, as in the "honey" and the "matters" mentioned in Proverbs, but the *extent*. When we lack self-control, we become gluttonous, wasteful of our time and resources, and further away from the Christ we Christians long to resemble.

Consider your behaviors thus far on your fasting journey: are you living excessively in other areas of your life right now? Or are you filling up on Daniel-Fast-friendly foods throughout the day to the point where you're not really hungry anymore?

Fasting demands that we have physical reminders of our hunger and our discomfort so that we are drawn to rely on Jesus. Ask God to point out what parts of your life are the "too much honey" so that you don't become the person "like a city whose walls are broken through."

*Dear Lord, I want to bear the fruits of Your spirit and my heart desires to be more like Jesus. Show me where I am lacking in self-control and help me to see where I am living in excess. Grant me the strength to exert self-control over these areas so that I might know Your peace.*

## Day 13: Think About These Things

Philippians 4: 8-9 (NIV)

*Finally, brothers, whatever is true, whatever is honorable, whatever is just, whatever is pure, whatever is lovely, whatever is commendable, if there is any excellence, if there is anything worthy of praise, think about these things. What you have learned and received and heard and seen in me—practice these things, and the God of peace will be with you.*

Does it ever seem to you that when we are finally free to break away from the rest of our hectic days for some quiet time with the Lord that it's far from quiet?  We saddle Him with requests, tears, and our rambling words—all of this is fine with Him and yes, He wants us to bring to him all of our prayers and worries.  However, how often are we able to be still before the Lord and just reflect on His goodness and love?

It can be quite the challenge to stop our tongues from wagging and hold tight, basking in His glory for however brief the moments may be.  In his letter to the church at Philippi, however, the apostle Paul encourages us to "practice these things," namely, thinking about "whatever is true, whatever is noble..." as the verse says.

On days where you may not know how to begin your time with God, don't worry about what you "have to say." Instead, follow Paul's suggestion. Think about what is true, honorable, just, pure, lovely, commendable, excellent, and praiseworthy. These may be things you observe in your daily world, or they may be certain characteristics of the Lord that you especially admire as of late. Soon enough, you will find that peace replaces the hectic aspects of your day.

*Dear Lord, thank You for all of the goodness surrounding me. Help me to see more of it in my day-to-day life. Remind me that when I see things that are true, honorable, pure, lovely, excellent, and praiseworthy, that they are all reflections of some aspect of Your Holiness.*

## Day 14: Being Still Before The Lord

Psalm 46: 10 (NIV)

*He says, "Be still, and know that I am God;*
*I will be exalted among the nations,*
*I will be exalted in the earth."*

There is an element in the original Quaker tradition that calls for a time of collective meditation, or group silence. What happens is that the congregation sits together, without uttering a word, and each member has the chance to pray, meditate, or otherwise reflect on God and who He is.

While it's not necessarily easy to sit in collective silence, we think it's much easier than sitting still before the Lord when we're on our own—after all, there's an entire group of people around us, who know us, and there's some strange sense of accountability there, when our accountability to the Lord should be enough.

You might be afraid to sit still before the Lord because you don't know what to do. Maybe you're scared to try it because you think you might fall asleep.
Perhaps you have so much on your heart that you want to share with Him that you don't see the need to be still.

When we are calm, quiet, alone, and still before God, we are focusing our minds and hearts directly on Him. We don't bring our words; we don't bring our requests. It is during this very quiet, personal time that we can reflect on who God really is. It is He who can part the oceans; it is He who can calm the storm; it is He who can walk on the water. It is God and God alone who will be exalted among all the nations.

In these very small, quiet moments, we allow God to show us just how big and powerful He really is.

*Dear Lord, I praise you because of who You are, the one true God of all the nations. Help me to be still and focused on Your power and might so that I can know you more.*

## Day 15: Being God's Captive

Joshua 1: 8-9 (ESV)

*This Book of the Law shall not depart from your mouth, but you shall meditate on it day and night, so that you may be careful to do according to all that is written in it. For then you will make your way prosperous, and then you will have good success. Have I not commanded you? Be strong and courageous. Do not be frightened, and do not be dismayed, for the Lord your God is with you wherever you go.*

Have you ever had something take your thoughts captive? Surely you have. There have probably been nights where you've tossed and turned over the events of the day, or because of the anxiety you feel about what might happen tomorrow. On the other hand, if you've ever been lovesick, you know that your days tend to go like some of the songs on the radio, where you think about your new love interest 24/7 and can't wait for them to call.

This passage from Joshua tells us that God wants our thoughts. He wants to hold our thoughts captive. He wants to be the one we think about night and day—and He promises that this is the path towards prosperity. Since none of us are born with a blueprint for how life should, we should consider that the best chance for happiness and success that we have is with God.

Fasting provides excellent opportunities to consume the word of God throughout the day. Each meal presents an opportunity to thank God for His provision; each pang of hunger reminds us of Him.

*Dear Lord, I want to feast on Your word and grow in the knowledge of You. I trust in Your plan to lead me to into goodness. Nourish my spirit with Your truth and help me to feast on it throughout my day.*

## Day 16: Cravings

1 Peter 2: 1-3

*Therefore, rid yourselves of all malice and all deceit, hypocrisy, envy, and slander of every kind. Like newborn babies, crave pure spiritual milk, so that by it you may grow up in your salvation, now that you have tasted that the Lord is good.*

Any time you give something up, you notice that you may have a craving for it even more than you did before. The old adage, "you always want what you can't have" rings true at times. It can take awhile for cravings to go away. At this point in your fast, you may have noticed that your cravings are dissipating and that you are growing *slightly* more comfortable with your new eating habits.

Cravings don't have to be bad, however. They can certainly be used for good, as Peter reminds us. We are instructed to "crave pure spiritual milk" once we know that the "Lord is good."

One way to develop this kind of craving is to do the exact opposite of what you are doing on your fast right now: don't give it up! The more time you spend with God, the more you'll want to be with Him. The more you study the Bible, the more you'll want to know. And the more you know Jesus, the more you'll be like Him.

*Dear Lord, help me to stay away from the sinful nature of deceit, hypocrisy, envy, and slander by giving me a craving for You.  Nourish my spirit with Your purity and  goodness so that I may grow closer to you.*

## Day 17: Worship

Isaiah 29:13 (GW)

*The Lord says: "These people come near to me with their mouth and honor me with their lips, but their hearts are far from me. Their worship of me is made up of rules made by humans."*

When we think of the term "worship," a myriad of images may come to mind. You might picture a man on his knees in prayer, a service filled with music, or an opulent cathedral decked out in stained glass. The idea of worship conjures a different scene from person to person.

Some churches promise "an awesome worship experience" and "a great worship experience" at their Sunday morning services. Friends are known to leave church saying "worship was amazing today!" or "I couldn't get into the music this morning and I couldn't worship."

Is this what worship has become?

Somewhere along the way, churches and believers concocted various notions about what was considered *worship* and *worshipful* and what was not. Have you fallen into the trap of going through the motions, saying the right things, and using current church lingo? Have you ever felt that your best efforts towards worshipping God weren't enough?

The word *worship* means to bow oneself down in reverence or honor, plain and simple. Participating wholeheartedly in the Daniel Fast is an act of worship in itself. When we seek to worship God, we are making ourselves humble and lowering our heads to acknowledge the presence and power of The Almighty. It is our responsibility and our responsibility alone to meet God at His feet and worship the King of Kings. When we have hearts that yearn to praise our Maker, worship begins.

*Dear Lord, create in me a desire to bow at Your holy feet in worship. Draw my heart close to yours. Teach me to worship you in purity and in truth.*

## Day 18: The Big Box

Philippians 4:19 (NASB)

*And my God will supply all your needs according to His riches in glory in Christ Jesus.*

The invention of the big-box store has served as a boon to many smaller mom-and-pop businesses, certainly, but nobody can deny the sheer convenience of shopping at discount clubs or the "mart of the moment." Where else can you purchase eggs, batteries, Christmas decorations, a new coat, and the latest best seller under one roof—and all for a discount? Many families take advantage of big-box benefits, since all of their needs can be met in one swift drive to the store and back.

Paul shares with us how Jesus not only carries more character than the big box store, but how He is the supplier who can meet all of our needs. He is the Author of our faith, the Comforter, the Commander, the Counselor, the Faithful Witness, the Guide, the Hope, the Judge, the Mediator, the Prince of Peace, the Redeemer, the Rock, the Savior, and the Way.

Today, take time to reflect on the many names we call God. Who is He showing Himself to be in your life during this time of fasting?

*Dear Lord, thank you for all that You are. You know my needs and my desires, and I know that you are the Great Supplier who will meet all of my needs. Reveal Yourself to me as I continue my final days of fasting.*

## Day 19: Serving The Boss

1 Samuel 12: 24 (NASB)

*Only fear the Lord and serve Him in truth with all your heart; for consider what great things He has done for you.*

Have you ever had to work for a boss that you didn't get along with?

Maybe you had opposing personalities; maybe you questioned his or her leadership; maybe that boss was unhappy and took it out on all of the employees. It can be difficult to do your best work for a boss that you don't connect with on a professional level.

Likewise, when we feel that our boss is fair and just and treats us with respect, we are much more inclined to produce some of our greatest work.

As Christians, we work to serve the Boss, all right. As humans, we are sometimes angry with Him if things don't go our way—but His ways are always higher and better than our own. We are likely to praise Him in good times; we tend to turn away in the bad times—when we should especially seek His counsel. We are blessed that this Boss grants us grace and forgiveness, but He doesn't give us a break from our one job: serving Him honestly and wholeheartedly.

During the fast, you may have felt like taking a break, especially since the end seemed so far away. (Well done, brothers and sisters—you're almost there.) However, staying steadfast with your Daniel Fast diet and seeking God's face numerous times a day is what God has called you to do during this time.

Even though the fast is ending in a short while, this period of worship, prayer, and service doesn't need. Today, ask God how you can serve Him in the days after the fast.

*Dear Lord, I praise You for who You are and thank You for all that You have done for me. Continue to inspire my heart towards serving You wholly and honestly. Guide me to ways that I can continue to serve you when my time of fasting ends.*

## Day 20: Crossing The Finish Line

2 Corinthians 7:1 (NASB)

*Therefore, having these promises, beloved, let us cleanse ourselves from all defilement of flesh and spirit, perfecting holiness in the fear of God.*

At times, fasting can feel like running a 5K—or even a marathon: you set your eyes on the finish line, and when you get through, you're clearly exhausted. However, you may have noticed that when someone finally crosses the finish line they keep on running for a little while. So should we be when it comes to ending our fast.

That's not to suggest that you continue to eat from a restricted diet from now until the end of time; however, we should remain mindful of *all* of our habits from this point forward—eating habits included.

You have nearly completed three weeks of fasting—and three weeks of intense prayer, study, and worship. The whole act of fasting is an act of worship, essentially. Hopefully you have not only become healthier, but you have developed a keener sense of who you are in Christ and who God is to you.

Because of this commitment, we should be wary about introducing old habits into our new lifestyle—our new, *improved* lifestyle that is more centered on God than ever before. As Paul writes to the church in Corinth, "let us cleanse ourselves from all defilement of flesh and spirit."

You know about God's promises. You have a clear vision of who God is. It should be impossible to move on to the next stage of life knowing these things while resuming old ways, but temptation can be strong. As the Daniel Fast approaches its end, take some time to ask God to reinforce the lessons you've learned along the way the past few weeks.

*Dear Lord, thank You for Your promises to me and for your revelations. Help me to stay close to you as my time of fasting ends. Give me the strength and perseverance I need to continue walking closely with You.*

## Day 21: Mind Renewal

Romans 12: 1-2

*Therefore, I urge you, brothers and sisters, in view of God's mercy, to offer your bodies as a living sacrifice, holy and pleasing to God—this is your true and proper worship. Do not conform to the pattern of this world, but be transformed by the renewing of your mind. Then you will be able to test and approve what God's will is—his good, pleasing and perfect will.*

Every now and then, a pop-up will appear on your computer screen reminding you that a piece of software has expired and it's time to renew the license if you're going to continue using that program.

How many of us address that issue immediately? Probably very few. The pop-ups are a good reminder, but they tend to become a nuisance until we finally go ahead and fill in all the information and fork over our credit cards to renew the license.

Through this fast, you have done what Paul encouraged the Romans to do: "offer your body as a living sacrifice." This act of worship has hopefully drawn you closer to God and He has been at work, revealing things about Himself and His plan for you.

Each day of this fast has been like a pop-up on the computer screen, reminding you to renew your license; however, the nature of the Daniel Fast itself refuses to let you minimize the screen. Instead, you are consistently being challenged and presented with opportunities to dwell on the things of God.

Though your time of fasting is drawing to a close, do not forget all that you have learned over this course of time—rather follow the words of Paul and "be transformed by the renewing of your mind." Has God used this fast to reveal to you His perfect will? Has He clearly closed doors and opened others? Has He spoken to the small corners of your heart over issues that only He would know to address? *Do not conform to the pattern of this world, but be transformed by the renewing of your mind.*

*Dear Lord, thank you for using this fast to teach me more about You, Your ways, and Your perfect will. Thank you for renewing my mind and revealing to me Your truth. Continue to transform me into who You want me to become.*

# Breakfast

## Currant and Almond Toasted Muesli

3 c. old-fashioned oats
½ c. water
2 ½ T. vegetable oil
½ c. raw almonds
½ c. sunflower seeds
¼ c. sesame seeds
½ c. unsweetened flaked coconut
1 c currants, unsweetened
4 peaches
unsweetened soy milk

1. Preheat oven to 325.
2. Place all ingredients through blueberries in a large bowl and mix well.
3. Line a baking tray with foil and spread the mixture evenly over the foil.
4. Bake for 30 minutes, stirring occasionally, until lightly browned.
5. Let cool and add currants and peaches.
6. Serve with unsweetened soy milk.

Makes 4 1-cup servings of muesli

Nutritional information (for muesli): 543 calories, 29.9g fat, 5mg sodium, 61.1g carbohydrates, 12.6g fiber, 13g sugar, 14.4g protein

## Stuffed Breakfast Squash

2 2-lb. acorn squash, unpeeled
1/2 cup quinoa
1 1/2 cups water
1 cup chopped apple
1 teaspoon ground cinnamon
1/4 teaspoon ground cloves
1/4 teaspoon nutmeg
1/4 cup chopped pecans
1/4 cup chopped dates
1/4 cup chopped apricots
1/4 cup golden raisins
1/4 cup unsweetened coconut

1. Preheat oven to 375 degrees.
2. Cut squash in half lengthwise and remove seeds. Place halves, cut side down, in a large baking dish. Pour in enough water to bring water to about 1/4-inch deep. Bake 40 minutes.
3. In the meantime, heat quinoa, water, apples, cinnamon, cloves, and nutmeg in a small saucepan; bring to a boil.
4. Reduce heat to low, and cover. Simmer gently with lid tilted for 20 minutes or until most of the liquid is absorbed.
5. Stir in pecans and raisins, and set aside
6. Fill each squash half with 1/2 cup apple-quinoa mixture and bake for an additional 10 minutes.
7. Sprinkle with coconut and serve warm.

Makes 4 servings (1 serving = 1/2 squash with 1/2 cup filling)

Nutritional information: 399 calories, 8.4g fat, 20mg sodium, 82.8g carbohydrate, 11.7g fiber, 16.6g sugar, 8g protein

## Baked Quinoa

1/2 cup quinoa
3/4 cup almond meal
1/2 cup rolled oats
1/2 cup unsweetened coconut (plus additional for sprinkling)
1 tsp. cinnamon
1/4 tsp. ground ginger
1/8 tsp. allspice
1/2 tsp. salt
3/4 c. almond milk
1/4 c. unsweetened applesauce
1 c. blueberries
2 peaches, diced

1. Preheat oven to 350 degrees.
2. Mix dry ingredients together.
3. In a separate bowl, mix wet ingredients.
4. Pour the wet ingredients into the dry ingredients; stir well.
5. Spread fruit on bottom of an 8x8 baking dish. Spoon the quinoa mixture over fruit.
6. Bake for 30 minutes or until golden and bubbly.
7. Serve warm with a sprinkle of coconut.

Makes about 6 1/2-cup servings

Nutritional information: 268 calories, 8.9g fat, 201mg sodium, 26.6g carbohydrate, 5.7g fiber, 8.1g sugar, 6.7g protein

## Peanut Butter Cakes

8 plain brown rice cakes
1/2 c. natural peanut butter, divided
1 banana, sliced
1/4 c. raisins

1. Spread 2 TB. peanut butter over one side of each rice cake.
2. Top with banana slices and raisins.

Makes 4 servings (1 serving = 2 cakes with topping)

Nutritional information: 393 calories, 17.2g fat, 125mg sodium, 49.3g carbohydrate, 4.6g fiber, 11.3g sugar, 13.6g protein

## Breakfast Burritos

1 banana, diced
1/2 c. strawberries, chopped
3/4 c. natural nut butter
1/2 c. unsweetened coconut
4 whole-wheat tortillas

1. Combine all ingredients except for tortillas. Mix well.
2. Fill each tortilla with nut butter and fruit mixture.

Makes 2 servings (1 serving = 2 tortillas)

Nutritional information: 420 calories, 28.2g fat, 22mg sodium, 29.4g carbohydrate, 7.6g fiber, 8.3g sugar, 17.2g protein

# Lunch Recipes

### Veggie Delight
16 oz. package shredded cabbage
1 c. carrots, peeled and grated
½ c. broccoli, chopped
½ c. cherry tomatoes, halved
½ c. celery, sliced
½ c. cucumber, peeled and diced
1/3 c. olive oil
2 T. vinegar
1 T. mustard
1 tsp. garlic salt

1. Combine vegetables in a large salad bowl.
2. Whisk together remaining ingredients; pour over vegetables.
3. Toss to coat.

Makes 4 1/2-cup servings

Nutritional information: 184 calories, 17.8g fat, 0 cholesterol, 36m sodium, 6.6g carbohydrates, 2.1g fiber, 2.6g sugar, 1.8g protein

## Sunflower Strawberry Salad

2 c. strawberries, hulled and sliced
1 apple, cored and diced
1 c. green seedless grapes, halved
½ c. celery, thinly sliced
¼ c. raisins
1 T. sunflower seeds
lettuce leaves

1. Combine all ingredients except for sunflower seeds.
2. Cover and chill for 1 hour.
3. Sprinkle with seeds and spoon over lettuce leaves.

Makes 6 ½ c. servings

Nutritional Information: 74 calories, 0.4g fat, 0 cholesterol, 13mg sodium, 18.2g carbohydrate, 5.1g fiber, 13.7g sugar, 0.7g protein

## Garlic and Tomato Soup

3 large tomatoes, cubed
2 bell peppers, diced
10 cloves garlic, coarsely chopped, divided
½ c. olive oil
2 c. water
1 tsp. salt
black pepper to taste

1. Combine tomatoes, peppers, and half of the garlic in a food processor; pulse until tomatoes are chopped, set aside.
2. Heat oil in a saucepan over medium heat. Add tomato mixture and cook, stirring often, for 5-10 minutes.
3. Add remaining ingredients and bring to a boil.
4. Reduce heat to low and simmer for 10 minutes.

Makes (4) 1 ½ c. servings

Nutritional Information: 270 calories, 25.7g fat, 595mg salt, 11.4g carbohydrate, 3.1g fiber, 6.1g sugar, 2.3g protein

## Roasted Broccoli and Asparagus

2 T. extra virgin olive oil
1/2 c. broccoli, chopped
1/2 c. asparagus, chopped
juice of 1 lemon
kosher salt and pepper

1. Preheat oven to 425 degrees.
2. Place broccoli and asparagus pieces in a baking dish.
3. Drizzle with olive oil and lemon juice.
4. Add salt and pepper to taste.
5. Mix well and roast for 425 for 25 minutes or until tender.

Makes 1 (1-cup) serving

Nutritional information: 288 calories, 28.2g fat, 16mg sodium, 5.5g carbohydrate, 2.6g fiber, 2g sugar, 2.7g protein.

## Marinated Vegetable Salad

1 can carrots, drained
1 can wax beans, drained
1 can red kidney beans, drained
1 can chickpeas, drained
1 can French green beans, drained
1 can black beans, drained
1 can corn, drained
1/3 c. vinegar
2 T. vegetable oil
1/2 tsp. caraway seed
salt and pepper to taste

1. Rinse all ingredients in a colander and drain well.
2. In a separate bowl, combine vinegar, vegetable oil, caraway seed, salt and pepper.
3. Pour over vegetables and chill in refrigerator to marinate (at least 4 hours).
4. Serve cold or at room temperature.

Makes 8 (3/4-cup) servings

Nutritional information: 618 calories, 8.1g fat, 221mg sodium, 107.6g carbohydrate, 27.1g fiber, 12.2g sugar, 33.7g protein

## Asian Spinach Salad

2 9-oz. bags of baby spinach
1/3 c. crushed sesame seeds
3-4 T. soy sauce

1. Boil the spinach for 2 minutes.
2. Rinse with cold water and squeeze out the water.
3. Chop into small pieces.
4. In a medium bowl, stir together soy sauce and sesame seeds.
5. Add spinach to the bowl and mix well.

Makes 2 (1-cup) servings

Nutritional information: 71 calories, 1554mg sodium, 11.1g carbohydrate, 5.8g fiber, 1.5 sugar, 8.8g protein

## Spicy Black Bean Burgers

1 (15-ounce) can black beans, rinsed and drained
1 large sweet potato, cooked
¼ cup brown rice flour
½ tablespoon dried parsley
¼ teaspoon chipotle chile pepper seasoning
¼ teaspoon garlic powder
¼ teaspoon salt
1/8 tsp. cumin
1/8 tsp. onion powder
1/8 teaspoon pepper
olive oil
Slices of red onion, tomatoes, spinach

1. Preheat oven to broil setting.
2. In a large bowl, mash black beans and sweet potato.
3. Mix in brown rice flour, parsley, chipotle seasoning, garlic powder, onion powder, cumin, salt, and pepper.
4. Brush a baking sheet with olive oil.
5. Working in 1/3 c. increments, flatten and shape bean mixture into small flat disks. Press down with a spatula.
6. Broil 4 inches from heat about 7 minutes or until golden brown. Flip burgers with spatula. Broil 2 more minutes.
7. Serve with red onion, tomato, and spinach leaves.

Makes 6 servings (1 serving = 1 bean burger)

Nutritional information: 294 calories, 1.9g fat, 112mg sodium, 55.6g carbohydrate, 12.1g fiber, 3.5g sugar, 16.4g protein

## Italian-style Rice and Beans

1/2 T. extra-virgin olive oil
1/2 c. chopped onion
1 clove garlic, minced
1 (28-ounce) can crushed tomatoes
1 (15.5-ounce) can cannellini beans, rinsed and drained
1 T. chopped fresh basil or 1 teaspoon dried basil
1 tsp. fennel seed
1 T. chopped fresh parsley or 1 teaspoon dried parsley
1/2 tsp. salt
1/8 tsp. pepper
4 cups cooked brown rice

1. Heat olive oil over medium heat in a large skillet.
2. Add onions and garlic, cooking until soft and golden.
3. Stir in remaining ingredients.
4. Cook over low heat for 30 minutes.
5. Serve ½ cup rice topped with ½ cup beans.

Makes 8 servings

Nutritional information: 578 calories, 3.9g fat, 355mg sodium, 114.2g carbohydrate, 20.4g fiber, 7.1g sugar, 22.6g protein

.

## Squash and Fennel Soup

1. T. olive oil
1/2 fennel bulb, sliced
2 shallots, chopped,
1 apple, chopped
2-1/2 cups cooked squash
3 c. vegetable broth
1 T. lemon juice
salt and pepper to taste

1. In a saucepot, heat oil over medium heat.
2. Cook fennel bulb, shallots, and apple in oil until tender.
3. In a blender or with an immersion blender, add squash, 1 c. broth, and apple mixture, blending until smooth.
4. Add remaining ingredients and simmer on low 10-15 minutes.

Makes 4 (1 cup) servings

Nutritional information: 102 calories, 4.7g fat, 594mg sodium, 11.1g carbohydrate, 2.6g fiber, 6.3g sugar, 4.7g protein

## Spring Salad

2 c. thawed frozen peas
4 radishes, diced
1 can of water chestnuts
1/2 c. diced hearts of palm
1 1/2 tsp. onion powder
1 tsp. vinegar
salt and pepper to taste.

1. Combine all ingredients in a large bowl, coating well.

Makes 2 (1 cup) servings

Nutritional information: 19 calories, 160mg sodium, 3.5g carbohydrate, 1.1g fiber, 1.2g protein

## Shining Carrot Soup

2 tsp. olive oil
1 large onion, chopped
3 stalks celery, chopped
2 cloves garlic, chopped
4 c. sliced carrots
1 tsp. Italian seasoning
1 tsp. dried basil
1 qt. vegetable broth
salt and pepper to taste

1.  Heat the olive oil in a large pot over medium heat.
2.  Add all ingredients through broth and cook for 10 minutes or until tender.
3.  Pour in the vegetable broth, cover, and simmer for 25 minutes or until the carrots are tender.
4.  Blend with an immersion blender or by pouring ladles into a stand blender.
5.  Season with salt and pepper.

Makes 6 (1-cup) servings

Nutritional information: 111 calories, 6g fat, 567mg sodium, 10.6g carbohydrate, 2.7g fiber, 5.2g sugar, 4.3g protein

## Moo Shu Vegetables

2 tsp. sesame oil
3 scallions, thinly sliced
3 c. thinly sliced bok choy or kale
1 red bell pepper, thinly sliced
2 carrots, thinly sliced
3/4 c. thinly sliced mushrooms
3/4 c. bean sprouts
1 block tofu, crumbled
3 tsp. grated fresh ginger
2 cloves garlic, minced
2 T. soy sauce

1. In a large skilled over medium-high heat, heat oil.
2. Add all ingredients through tofu. Saute for 3-4 minutes.
3. Add remaining ingredients and cook until sprouts are soft (about 2-3 minutes).

Makes 6 (1/2 cup) servings

Nutritional information: 75 calories, 2.5g fat, 334mg sodium, 10.1g carbohydrate, 2.4g fiber,2.3g sugar, 4.7g protein

# Dinner

## Grilled Farmer's Market Veggies

3 zucchini, sliced ¾-inch thick
3 yellow squash, sliced 3/4 –inch thick
1 small eggplant, sliced 3/4 –inch thick
1 yellow or Vidalia onion, sliced 3/4 –inch thick
2 tomatoes, sliced 1-inch thick
½ c. balsamic vinegar
1 c. vegetable oil
2 cloves garlic, minced
1 T. fresh rosemary, minced
1 T. fresh oregano, chopped
1 T. fresh basil, chopped
1 T. fresh parsley, chopped
salt and pepper to taste

1. Combine vegetables in a large bowl.
2. In separate bowl, whisk together the remaining ingredients.
3. Pour the wet ingredients over the vegetables and toss to coat. Marinate at room temperature for an hour.
4. Remove vegetables from marinade using a slotted spoon. Arrange on a grill over medium-hot heat.
5. Grill 2-5 minutes on each side, basting with marinade, until tender.

Makes 6--1 ½ cup servings

Nutritional information: 396 calories, 15g fat, 0 cholesterol, 25 mg sodium, 15.6g carbohydrates, 6.2g fiber, 7.1g sugar, 3.9g protein

## Iowa Corn Soup

1 tsp. olive oil
½ c. onion, diced
1 clove garlic, minced
½ t. ground cumin
4 c. corn kernels (fresh or frozen)
2 new potatoes, diced
½ tsp. kosher salt
1/8 tsp. black pepper
4 c. vegetable broth
1 t. fresh cilantro, chopped

1. Heat oil in a large pot over medium heat.
2. Saute onion, garlic, and cumin until onion is tender and fragrant, about 5 minutes.
3. Add remaining ingredients through cilantro and bring to a boil.
4. Reduce heat to a simmer and cook until potatoes are tender, about 20 minutes.
5. Add cilantro, stir.

Makes (4) 2-cup servings

Nutritional information: 278 calories, 3.7g fat, 300mg sodium, 48.2g carbohydrate, 6.5g fiber, 6.6g sugar, 6g protein

## 7-Veggie Stew

1 3 lb. butternut squash, peeled, seeded, and cubed
2 c. eggplant, peeled and cubed
2 c. zucchini, diced
10-oz. package frozen okra, thawed
8-oz . can no-sugar-added tomato sauce
1 c. onion, chopped
1 tomato, chopped
1 carrot, peeled and thinly sliced
½ c. vegetable broth
1/3 c. raisins
1 clove garlic, chopped
½ tsp. ground cumin
½ tsp. turmeric
¼ tsp. red pepper flakes
¼ tsp. cinnamon
¼ tsp. paprika

1. Combine all ingredients in a slow cooker.
2. Cover and cook on LOW for 8-10 hours.

Makes 8 1 ½ c. servings

Nutritional information: 138 calories, 0.6g fat, 328g sodium, 33.4g carbohydrate, 6.8g fiber, 11.4g sugar, 3.6g protein

## Baked Beans

4 tsp. olive oil
1 onion, finely chopped
1 clove of garlic, crushed
1 tsp. fresh thyme, finely chopped
½ tsp. dried oregano
1 14-oz. can diced tomatoes, mashed
½ c. water
2 14-oz. cans cannellini beans, drained and rinsed
salt and pepper to taste

1. Preheat the oven to 325.
2. Heat the oil in a Dutch oven over medium heat.
3. Add onion; stir and cook until soft (about 5-10 minutes); add garlic, thyme, and oregano.
4. Add the tomatoes and water, bringing to a boil. Reduce heat to simmer and cook for 10 minutes.
5. Add the beans and stir. Cover the Dutch oven and bake for 30 minutes. Season with salt and pepper.

Makes 4 1 ½ c. servings

Nutritional information: 754 calories, 6.4g fat, 239mg sodium, 130g carbohydrates, 53.3g fiber, 11.1g sugar, 49.5g protein

## Mexican Casserole

2 T. vegetable oil
1 c. white corn kernels
1 c. yellow corn kernels
2 cloves garlic, minced
1 medium green pepper, chopped
1 medium onion, chopped
1 15-oz. can pinto beans, drained, rinsed, and mashed
½ tsp. garlic powder
½ tsp. onion powder
1 16-oz. can tomato sauce
1 c. salsa (no sugar added)
1 tsp. cumin
½ tsp. salt
1 pkg. small whole wheat tortillas
chopped cilantro and chopped green onions

1. Heat a large skillet over medium heat. Add vegetable oil and saute corn, garlic, pepper, and onion until tender.
2. Preheat oven to 350 degrees.
3. Add the remaining ingredients through salt to skillet; simmer for 15 minutes.
4. Spoon a small amount of skillet mixture to into the bottom of a 13x9 inch baking dish. Cover with a layer of tortillas. Continue alternating layers of vegetable mixture and

tortillas, making the final layer with remaining vegetable mixture.
5. Cover with foil and bake for 25 minutes. Sprinkle with cilantro and chopped green onions.

Make 6 1-cup servings

Nutritional Information: 352 calories, 5.9g fat, 860mg sodium, 59.5g carbohydrates, 14.2g fiber, 8.2g sugar, 18g protein

## Stuffed Cabbage

2 large onion, chopped
5 cloves of garlic, minced and divided
1 large can of crushed tomatoes
1 14-oz. can of tomato sauce
1 TB. tomato paste
¼ c. golden raisins
1 large head of cabbage
1 ¼ c. dry lentils, cooked to total 3 cups
2 T. fresh parsley, minced
2 T. fresh lemon juice
¼ tsp. allspice
salt and pepper to taste

1. Heat a large non-stick pan over medium heat and cook ½ of the onions until soft, about 5 minutes. Stir in ½ of the garlic and cook for another minute. Add all of the tomato-based ingredients and stir.
2. Reduce heat to low and cover, cooking for a half hour.
3. In the meantime, fill a large pan with enough water to cover a cabbage and bring it to a boil
4. Using a paring knife, cut the cabbage at an angle around the core and remove as much as you can. Put the cabbage core-end up into the boiling water and cook until the leaves soften.
5. Remove each leaf and repeat until you have 10-12 whole cabbage leaves

6. Place the leaves and the remaining cabbage head in a strainer and rinse under cold water. Finely shred the cabbage remaining on the head and add it to the sauce along with the raisins. Keep the sauce covered and continue to cook on at a low simmer.

7. In a medium bowl, mix the lentils and all remaining ingredients, adding salt and pepper to taste. Dry each cabbage leaf gently and trim the thick rib near the stem end of each leaf.

8. Put a cabbage leaf on your work surface with the stem towards you. Place about 1/3 cup of the lentil mixture near the stem end. Fold the stem over the filling and then fold the sides toward the middle. Roll the filling up the rest of the leaf. Repeat with remaining leaves.

9. Spread half of the tomato sauce in the bottom of a Dutch oven. Place each cabbage roll seam-side down. Spread the remaining sauce over the rolls.

10. Cover and cook on the lowest setting until the cabbage is tender, about 45-60 minutes, being careful not to burn the bottom.

Makes 6 servings (1 serving = 3 rolls)

Nutritional information: 171 calories, 352mg sodium, 36g carbohydrate,14.5g fiber, 9.3g sugar, 13.1g protein

## White Bean Chili

3 cans Great Northern beans, drained and rinsed
2 green peppers, chopped
1 jalapenos, minced
2 shallots, minced
2 cloves garlic, pressed
1 T. fresh cilantro
2 c. vegetable broth
1 c. corn
½ teaspoon cumin
½ teaspoon chili powder
salt and pepper to taste
chopped cilantro and lime wedges

1. In a food processor, puree 1 ½ cups of the beans. Place in a saucepot and set aside.
2. Add all remaining ingredients to the pot.
3. Bring to a boil, then reduce heat to simmer.
4. Cook for 30 minutes or until vegetables are tender.
5. Season with salt and pepper, garnish with lime wedges and chopped cilantro.

Makes 4 (1 ½ cup) servings

Nutritional information: 721 calories, 3.1g fat, 287mg sodium, 132.4g carbohydrate, 41.g fiber, 6.6g sugar, 46.3g protein

## "Carmelized" Lentils

3 c. water
1 c. dry lentils, sorted and rinsed
2 tsp. Creole seasoning
1 T. extra-virgin olive oil
1 c. sliced yellow or Vidalia onion
3 cups cooked brown rice

1. Place water and lentils in a small saucepan. Bring to a boil, and lower heat.
2. Stir in Creole Seasoning.
3. Cover, and simmer with lid tilted for 40-45 minutes or until lentils are softened.
4. In a large skillet, heat olive oil over medium-low heat.
5. Add onions, cooking 20-25 minutes and stirring occasionally until onions are soft and brown.
6. Top 1 c. brown rice with lentils and onion mixture.

Makes 6 (1/3 cup) servings

Nutritional information: 485 calories, 5.2g fat, 369mg sodium, 93.3g carbohydrate, 13.4g fiber, 1.4g sugar, 15.6g protein

## Standard Stir-Fry

1 T. extra-virgin olive oil
2 c. chopped broccoli
1 c. chopped carrots
½ c. chopped onion
2 T. low-sodium soy sauce
2 T. sesame oil
3 T. vinegar
1 clove garlic, minced
¼ teaspoon ground ginger
3 cups cooked brown rice
¼ cup toasted chopped walnuts
2 tablespoons chopped green onion

1. Heat olive oil in a large skillet over medium heat, and add broccoli, carrots, and onions.
2. Cook until vegetables are softened, about 5-7 minutes, stirring occasionally. Increase heat to medium high.
3. Add remaining ingredients. Cook another 5 minutes or until heated through, and serve.

Makes 4 (1 ¼ cup) servings

Nutritional Information: 694 calories, 19g fat, 481mg sodium, 117.3g carbohydrate, 7.7g fiber, 3.3g sugar, 14.8g protein

## Butternut Squash and Greens

2 tsp. olive oil
3 c. chopped and washed Swiss chard
1 1/2 c. cubed and roasted butternut squash
1/8 tsp. ground coriander
1/8 tsp. ground cumin
1/4 tsp. salt
2 T. chopped almonds
2 T. raisins

1. In a large skillet, heat of olive oil over medium heat.
2. Add coriander and cumin. Saute one minute or until fragrant.
3. Add chard and cook until wilted.
4. Add in butternut squash and stir gently.
5. Add in the salt, raisins and chopped almonds.

*May serve over any appropriate Daniel Fast grains.

Makes 4 (1 cup) servings

Nutritional Information:  90 calories, 4g fat, 208mg sodium, 11.4g carbohydrate, 2g fiber, 4.3g sugar, 1.8g protein

## Roasted Brussels Sprouts and Pomegranate Dressing

1 ¼ c. water
1 c. quinoa
1 lb. Brussels Sprouts
1 T. olive oil
zest of 4 clementines
juice of 1 clementine
½ c. unsweetened pomegranate juice
2 T. vinegar
¼ cup olive oil
½ tsp. garlic powder
salt and pepper to taste

1. Preheat the oven to 425 degrees.
2. In a medium pot, boil water and add quinoa; cover and cook for 15 minutes.
3. Add all clementine components.
4. Toss sprouts with oil on a baking sheet and bake for 15 minutes, until browned.
5. In a separate bowl, mix juice, vinegar, and seasonings.
6. Mix sprouts and quinoa, dress with dressing, serve warm.

Makes 4 (3/4 cup) servings

Nutritional information: 337 calories, 18.9 calories, 33mg sodium, 36.3 carbohydrate, 7.1g fiber, 2.6g sugar, 9.6g protein

## Fake-Out Minestrone

1 TB. olive oil
1 large onion, diced
2 cloves garlic, pressed
2 carrots, peeled and diced
1 stalk celery, diced
4 c. vegetable broth
1 large can crushed tomatoes
1 can green beans
1 zucchini, diced
1 bag baby spinach
1 can cannellini beans, drained and rinsed

1. In a large pot over medium heat, heat olive oil.
2. Saute onion, garlic, carrots, and celery until soft.
3. Add all remaining ingredients and cook until soft and heated through.

Makes 4 (2 cup) servings

Nutritional information: 562 calories, 6.2g fat, 1254mg sodium, 94.3g carbohydrate, 38.1g fiber, 19.6g sugar, 38g protein

## Baked Spaghetti Squash

3 lb. spaghetti squash, sliced in half lengthwise
½ c. dried lentils
1 c. vegetable broth
1 large onion, diced
3 cloves garlic, minced
8 oz. sliced mushrooms
½ of a 14 oz. block of soft tofu, chopped/diced
1½ T. low-sodium soy sauce
½ tsp. dried sage
¼ tsp. dried thyme
3 c. kale, chopped with ribs removed
salt and pepper to taste

1. Preheat oven to 375F.
2. Place the two squash halves, cut side-down, into a large baking dish. Bake for 30-40 minutes, or until soft.
3. In the meantime, bring the vegetable broth to a boil in a small pot over high heat. Add lentils; reduce heat to a simmer.
4. Cover (and cook for 20 minutes or until soft.
5. In a large, non-stick pan, heat the onion and garlic over medium heat, until the onions begin to clear.
6. Add mushrooms to the pan and sauté until soft.
7. Add tofu, soy sauce, sage, and thyme.
8. Stir together and bring to a simmer. Adjust the heat to medium-low and mix in kale. Stir in cooked lentils.

9. In a 8x8 sauté pan, add lentil mixture and squash, mixing well. Season with salt and pepper
10. Bake for 15-20 minutes or until golden.

Makes 4 (1 cup) servings

Nutritional information: 259 calories, 2.7g fat, 805mg sodium, 50g carbohydrate, 9.9g fiber, 3.5g sugar, 14.1g protein

## Indian Chickpeas

1 clove of garlic
1/2 tsp. peppercorns
1/2 tsp. coriander seeds
2 T. olive oil
1 T. curry powder
2 c. vegetable broth
2 c. sliced potatoes
2 c. sliced carrots
2 c. cauliflower florets
1 14-oz. can chopped tomatoes
1 14-oz. can unsweetened coconut milk
1 14-oz. can chickpeas, rinsed and drained
2 T. soy sauce
8 fresh basil leaves, chopped

1. Using a mortar and pestle, make a ground paste with the garlic, peppercorns and coriander seeds into a paste.
2. Heat the oil in a Dutch oven over medium heat. Add paste and cook until fragrant.
3. Add curry powder and cook an additional 3-4 minutes.
4. Add broth, potatoes and carrots and bring to a gentle simmer
5. Add remaining ingredients through basil and cook until vegetables are tender.
6. Serve over hot brown rice and garnish with basil leaves.

Makes 6 (1 ¼ cup) servings

Nutritional information: 523 calories, 25.4g fat, 623mg sodium, 61.1g carbohydrate, 17.3g fiber, 14.5g sugar, 18.9g protein

## Conclusion

We hope you successfully completed your 21-day Daniel Sugar Diet. That very first day of fasting will be a challenge, as will the days ahead, and the twenty-first day (or conclusion of the fast) might seem like it will never come. Remember the virtue of patience, and keep in mind that twenty-one days is just a blip on the radar map of life—it will go by quickly.

While this particular Daniel Diet will soon be a thing of your personal past, it does not mean it should be forgotten; on the contrary, the period of fasting will impact your life forever.

If you feel that this book has helped you, please feel free to leave a review to encourage others to take the same journey you have. Thank you and I wish you health, happiness, and peace.

Made in the USA
Columbia, SC
22 April 2025

56993486R00052